Introduction

Are you caring for a person who suffers from Alzheimer's disease, Parkinson's disease, stroke-related dementia or any of the other diseases that leave people with memory loss and confusion? Then this guide is for you.

Caring for a person with memory loss and confusion can sometimes be an overwhelming experience. This guide was created to give you a simple, easy to use reference – a place where you can get the answers you need, when you need them the most. The suggestions in this guide come from caregivers like you who have had to find solutions to the everyday challenges of caring for a person with brain impairment.

How to Use This Guide

This guide is organized into the key areas of caring for a person with memory loss and confusion. Each section provides simple tips on how to deal with the most common issues.

Take a few moments to read through the table of contents (on page 2) and skim through each of the sections. Then choose tips from the areas where you need the most help. For example, if the person you are caring for is having trouble sleeping, turn to the section on "Sleep Problems." You will find specific suggestions to help you both get the rest you need. In addition, please read the sections on "Taking Care of Yourself" and "Getting the Help You Need."

Table of Contents

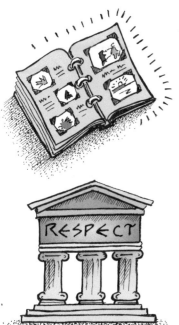

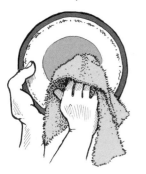

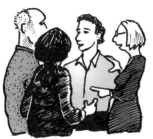

In memory of Arthur T. Bignell and his devotion to his wife, Helen.

About Memory Loss and Confusion

What Is Memory Loss and Confusion?

✓ Memory loss and confusion (also called dementia or brain impairment) is not a normal part of aging. It is the result of a medical disease or condition.
✓ There are many diseases that cause memory loss and confusion. Alzheimer's disease, stroke, Parkinson's disease and HIV-related dementia are a few.
✓ Other conditions that can also cause memory loss and confusion include reactions to medications, infections, and hearing or vision loss. These conditions may be treatable, so it is very important that the person you are caring for has had a complete medical evaluation.
✓ See a doctor who is knowledgeable about the causes of memory loss and confusion. Not all family physicians are.

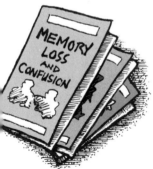

Learn About the Disease

✓ Learn as much as you can about the condition or disease that is causing the memory loss and confusion.
✓ Understanding the disease will help when you need to make caregiving and medical decisions.
✓ The person's doctor may be able to provide you with information. The library is another good resource. Look in the resources section of this book for other places to get information and help.

Plan for Daily Care

Set Routines and Schedules

✓ Having a routine or schedule will make life easier for you and the person for whom you are caring.

✓ Try going to bed, waking and eating meals at the same time each day.

✓ Set priorities. Plan the most difficult tasks for the person's best time of day.

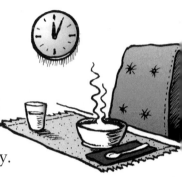

Plan with the Individual in Mind

✓ Remember that the person you are caring for has his or her own likes and dislikes.

✓ For example, some people with memory loss and confusion prefer quiet time. Others need to keep busy.

Prepare Ahead of Time

✓ Prepare as much of a task in advance as you can. At mealtimes, for example, have the food served before the person sits down at the table.

✓ Have the bath water ready and toothpaste on the toothbrush.

✓ Have clothes out and stacked in the order in which they will be put on.

Allow Plenty of Time

✓ Meals, bathing and other everyday tasks may take longer than they used to take.

✓ Leave extra time to get to appointments. Getting from one place to another may take more time too.

✓ Try not to rush. Rushing may create more confusion or anxiety Accidents happen more easily when people are rushed.

✓ Don't worry about being late. It is better to take your time.

Create a Calm Environment

✓ Limit the amount of change or distraction. Simple surroundings will make it less confusing for the person.
✓ Limit excessive noise from TV, loud music or talking.
✓ Keep counters clear and unnecessary items put away.
✓ Keep items used regularly in the same place.

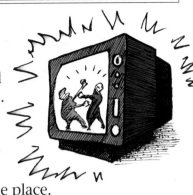

Be Flexible

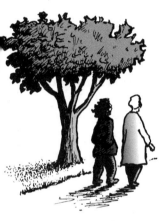

✓ Be ready to change plans if need be.
✓ Remember that the person's mental abilities can change from day to day, or even hour to hour. Adjust your expectations to match the person's abilities.
✓ If a certain activity is creating stress, try something else. For example, if the person isn't enjoying listening to music, try taking a walk instead.

Offer Plenty of Reassurance and Praise

✓ Praise and reassurance may help decrease the person's anxiety.
✓ Comments such as, "It's all right," may help the person feel calmer.
✓ Offer affection. Hold a hand or give a hug.

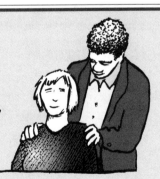

✓ Offer praise when the person is successful with a difficult task or activity.
✓ Remember to thank the person when he or she is able to help you.

Adapt Your Home for Safety

Focus On Prevention

✓ It's OK to make certain areas of the house "off limits" to the person with memory loss and confusion. Put locks on doors to prevent the person from visiting those areas.

✓ Don't leave the person home alone – even for a few minutes – if he or she can't respond to an emergency situation.

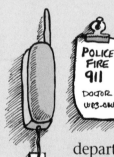

Have an Emergency Plan

✓ Remember that you can't always avoid accidents. Have a plan for fire and other types of emergencies – just in case.

✓ Post the plan near the phone with numbers for the police, fire department, poison control and doctor. Include the phone numbers of friends, family members or neighbors you can call for help too.

If the person you are caring for wanders, see page 23 of this guide for additional safety tips.

Check for Hazards

✓ Check every room for potential hazards.

✓ Remove clutter and put away items that may cause confusion. For example, don't leave the shaving cream next to the toothpaste.

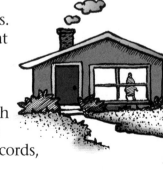

✓ Keep walkways, halls and paths through the house clear. Move tripping hazards such as low furniture. Secure electrical cords, phone cords and loose rugs.

✓ Lock up all poisons, medicines, cleaning products and insecticides. Lock up all sharp objects such as knives or razors.

Use Safety Devices

✓ Lock or secure all upstairs windows and doors that lead to balconies. Put gates at the top and bottom of stairways.

✓ Install safety latches or locks on cabinets where dangerous or breakable items are stored.

✓ Cover outlets not in use with safety covers.

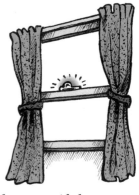

✓ Use door alarms or motion detectors to alert you if the person wanders outside or into an off-limits area.

Provide Good Lighting

✓ Make sure the house is well-lit. Light dark hallways and corners.

✓ Make sure lamps and light fixtures are secure and cannot be easily knocked over.

✓ Put nightlights in bathrooms, hallways and bedrooms.

✓ Provide lighting that can be reached and turned on easily.

Make the Bedroom Safe

✓ Clear closets and drawers of clutter.

✓ Remove or fasten down area rugs to prevent slipping in the night.

✓ Make sure there is a clear path to the bathroom or provide a bedside commode.

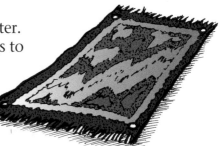

Create a Safe Bathroom

✓ Put away or lock up all items in the bathroom except essentials such as soap, towel, toothbrush and toothpaste.

✓ Use nonslip decals or mats in the tub and shower.

✓ Use nonskid rugs or mats to prevent slipping on a wet floor.

✓ Install grab bars in the shower or tub and around the toilet.

✓ Remove or disable locks on bathroom doors so that the person does not accidentally lock him or herself in the bathroom.

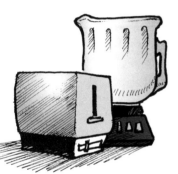

Secure the Kitchen

✓ Remove stove and oven knobs when not in use, or use childproofing devices.

✓ Remove or lock up all sharp kitchen utensils.

✓ Put away kitchen appliances such as blenders and toasters.

✓ Unplug the garbage disposal.

Prevent Burns

✓ Put guards around radiators and other heaters.

✓ Make sure the temperature gauge on the hot water heater is turned to 120 degrees or lower to prevent scalding.

✓ If the person smokes, supervise cigarettes and matches. Do not let the person smoke in bed.

✓ Or, put the cigarettes out of sight. The person may soon forget about smoking.

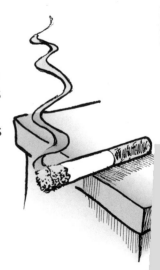

Keys to Better Communication

Treat the Person with Respect

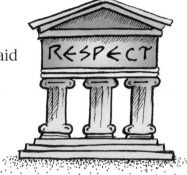

✓ Sometimes people with memory loss have trouble understanding what is said and communicating what they need.

✓ Although some illnesses make people behave in a childlike manner, remember that the person is an adult. Always talk to the person in a respectful manner.

✓ Don't talk about the person as if he or she isn't there.

Get the Person's Attention

✓ Using the person's first name to get his or her attention may help.

✓ Talk in a gentle, relaxed and matter-of-fact tone. Be sure to make eye contact.

✓ Try a gentle touch on the arm if the person isn't looking at you or can't see you. Let the person touch you too.

Use Short, Simple Sentences

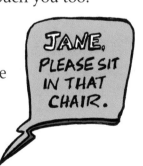

✓ Keep sentences short and easy to understand. For example, "Jane, please sit in that chair."

✓ Say each sentence slowly and clearly. If the person doesn't understand, try repeating what you said using the same words.

✓ Pause between sentences to give the person time to understand what has been said and time to respond.

Reduce Distractions

✓ Check for physical distractions such as glare from a window.

✓ Make sure the person is using his or her glasses or hearing aid.

✓ Reduce distracting noise or activity such as TV or loud music.

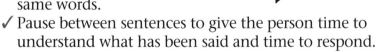

Use Concrete Words and Phrases

✓ Be specific. Say, "Here is your toast," instead of, "It's time for breakfast."

✓ Limit the number of choices in a question. For example, ask, "Would you like a glass of orange juice?" instead of, "What would you like to drink?"

✓ If the person does not seem to understand the meaning of a certain word, try another word that has the same meaning.

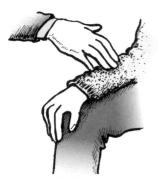

Use Signals Other Than Words

✓ Try waving or gently touching a person's arm to say hello.

✓ Smile or nod to show you understand what he or she is saying.

✓ Motion with your hand to invite the person to join you in an activity.

✓ Show the person what you want. Try pointing to something in addition to naming it.

✓ Label frequently used items and photos. A picture of a toilet on the door of the bathroom is often helpful.

Pay Attention to What Is Really Being Said

✓ Try to understand the meaning behind what the person is saying. For example, "I want to go home," may mean, "I'm anxious and need reassurance," or "I need to go to the bathroom."

✓ Look and listen for clues in behavior to determine what the person needs or wants. Pay attention to facial expressions and body language.

✓ Repeat back what you hear. For example, "You're hungry now, aren't you?"

✓ Pay attention to your body language too! Even if the person doesn't understand what you are saying, he or she may still be able to sense anger, frustration, pleasure or approval.

Everyday Activities

Adapt Daily Tasks

✓ When you provide activities, keep in mind the person's needs and likes.
✓ Change activities to fit the person's current abilities. Sometimes abilities change from day to day.
✓ Simple household chores such as folding towels, drying dishes or sweeping can be comforting for a person with memory loss and confusion.
✓ If the person has trouble remembering how to do a task, try showing him or her by doing it yourself first.
✓ Skills from the distant past will be remembered the longest.

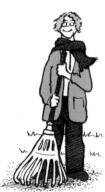

Modify Hobbies

✓ A person who played the piano may like listening to piano music.
✓ A gardener may still be able to rake leaves.
✓ Someone who cooked may still like to mash potatoes, shell peas or wash vegetables.

Provide Mental Stimulation

✓ Help the person think about the past. Look through photo albums, watch old movies or listen to music from the past.
✓ Provide simple tasks to stimulate the person's brain. Have the person separate checkers into red and black piles.
✓ Try reading aloud or having the person read to you.
✓ Social interactions at home or at a day care center can be enjoyable and mentally stimulating.

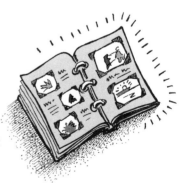

Exercise Daily

✓ Exercise may improve appetite and help with sleep problems. It also is a good outlet for excess energy and will help a person stay mobile.

✓ Schedule exercise for the person's most restless time of day.

✓ Take a daily walk, toss a beach ball or put on music and dance.

✓ Adapt sports. A person who played softball may enjoy a game of catch.

✓ For people with limited movement, try seated exercises or have them rock in a rocking chair.

✓ Remember that pacing and wandering in a safe environment can be a good source of exercise.

✓ Check with the person's doctor before beginning a new exercise routine.

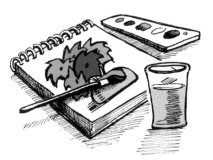

Encourage Self-Expression

✓ Try an art project such as painting or drawing.

✓ Knead, pound or flatten clay. Cut shapes with a cookie cutter.

✓ Have the person make a collage with shapes cut from colored paper.

Experiment!

✓ A person may enjoy a new activity or may no longer like old favorites.

✓ Don't insist on finishing a task. If the person becomes anxious during any activity, stop or change to a quiet or calming task.

✓ It is OK to provide busy work such as folding towels or winding yarn if it occupies or calms the person.

Make Bathing and Personal Care Easier

Monitor Grooming Needs

✓ Choose the person's most relaxed time of day for bathing and grooming.
✓ Monitor the person's bathing, teeth cleaning, hair care and skin care.
✓ Make sure finger nails and toe nails are trimmed weekly.

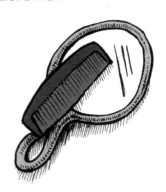

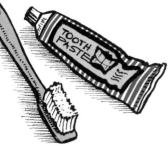

Brush Teeth Daily

✓ Help the person brush his or her teeth or clean dentures daily.
✓ Try brushing only the outside of the teeth if the person refuses to open his or her mouth.

Adapt Bathing

✓ A complete bath may not be necessary every day. A sponge bath is an alternative.
✓ Make sure the bathing area is warm and well lit. Always check the temperature of the bath or shower water.
✓ If a shower is upsetting, use a hand held shower or have the person take a bath instead.
✓ Use rubber mats to help reduce slipping in the bath. Make sure there are no puddles on the floor.
✓ Try handrails or a bath chair.

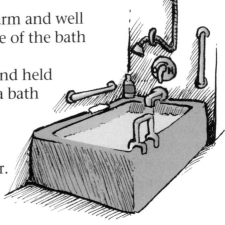

Help the Person Dress Appropriately

✓ Choose clothes and shoes that are easy to get on and off.
✓ Buy two of the same outfit if the person likes to wear the same thing every day.
✓ Choose clothing that fastens in the back for someone who repeatedly takes off his or her clothes.
✓ If the person wanders, choose brightly colored clothes that are easily seen.

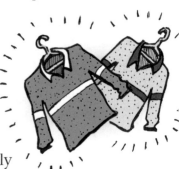

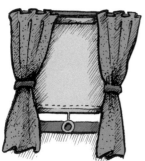

Treat the Person with Respect

✓ Many adults are embarrassed to have someone help them with bathing and grooming.
✓ Close doors and curtains for privacy. Wrap a towel around the person's shoulders while bathing.
✓ If the person is able to do a task, let him or her do it. Gently guide the person through each step. For example, give the person one piece of clothing at a time and tell them how to put it on.
✓ When you need to do something for the person, explain what you are doing. For example, "I'm going to brush your hair now"

Make Personal Care Simple and Safe

✓ Keep visible only those clothes that the person will be wearing.
✓ Eliminate accessories that can be put on wrong such as belts or scarves.
✓ Have the person's hair cut in a short, attractive style that needs minimal care.
✓ Remember that you may need to change your standards of grooming to fit the person's abilities.

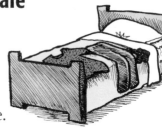

Tips for a Better Night's Sleep

Eliminate Alcohol and Caffeine

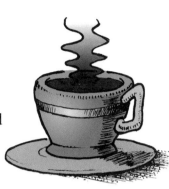

✓ Alcohol may disrupt sleep. Try serving nonalcoholic drinks such as juice.
✓ Offer nonalcoholic wine or beer.
✓ Caffeine can increase restlessness and interfere with sleep. Serve decaffeinated coffee instead of regular coffee.
✓ In addition to coffee, many foods and beverages such as chocolate, black tea and soft drinks have caffeine.

Prevent Daytime Napping

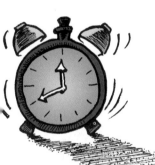

✓ Keep the person active and awake during the day. Make sure he or she gets exercise and is involved in daytime activities.
✓ If naps are necessary, keep them short and earlier in the day.
✓ Try to wake the person up earlier in the morning if he or she sleeps late.

Make Sure the Person Is Comfortable During the Night

✓ Adjust the room temperature and have extra blankets available.
✓ Make sure the person's bed, pillow and nightclothes are comfortable.
✓ Make sure the person isn't hungry or thirsty. Try a light snack such as toast before bedtime.
✓ Make sure the person uses the bathroom before bed.
✓ If the person is in pain, talk to a doctor about giving him or her pain medication (such as a non-aspirin pain reliever) at bedtime.

Create a Familiar Sleeping Area

✓ A favorite blanket or pillow may help the person relax.

✓ Use a nightlight to help the person know where he or she is.

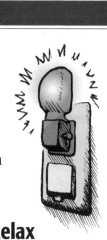

✓ Let the person sleep on the couch or in an armchair if he or she refuses to go to bed.

Help the Person Relax Before Bedtime

✓ Try playing soft music at bedtime.

✓ Avoid upsetting activities before bed. If taking a bath or putting on pajamas upsets the person, try doing those tasks earlier in the evening.

✓ You may even want to let the person sleep in comfortable clothes if changing into nightclothes is a problem.

Make It Safe In Case the Person Gets Up

✓ Keep the area around the bed clear. Make sure the path to the bathroom is softly but clearly lit.

✓ Put a commode next to the bed if finding the bathroom is a problem.

✓ If you sleep in a separate area of the house, use a room monitor (like those used for infants), a bed alarm, or a door alarm so that you can hear if the person gets up.

✓ Block stairs, secure doors and windows, and lock up dangerous items such as scissors and knives.

✓ If the person does get up, try gently guiding him or her back into bed. The person may have forgotten that it is time to sleep.

Make Mealtime Easier

Make Eating Easy

✓ Set a routine for when and where meals are served. Make mealtime a highlight of the day.
✓ Use bowls and spoons. They are often easier to handle than plates and forks.
✓ Use solid colored plates, tablecloths and place mats. They are less distracting than those with patterns.
✓ Fill glasses half full or use cups with non-spill lids. Try bendable straws.
✓ Use plastic dishes to reduce breakage and plastic aprons and tablecloths to make cleanup easier.

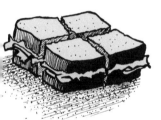

Serve Foods You Know the Person Likes

✓ Prepare foods in ways familiar to the person.
✓ If the person didn't like a food before, he or she probably won't like it now.
✓ Let the person have smaller, more frequent meals if that is what he or she wants.

Try Finger Foods

✓ It may be easier for the person to eat with his or her fingers instead of utensils.
✓ Offer foods that are easy to pick up such as cheese, small sandwiches or fresh fruits and vegetables.
✓ Always have the food cut up and ready to go when the person sits down to eat.
✓ Cut foods into small pieces to make it easier to chew and swallow.

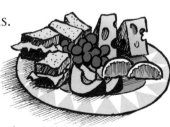

Check for Physical Comfort

✓ Test the temperature of the food. The person may not be able to tell you if the food is too hot or too cold.

✓ Check to see that the person is chewing food well. You may need to cut food into smaller pieces or puree it in a blender.

✓ Take the person to the dentist immediately if you suspect he or she is experiencing any pain while chewing.

✓ Make sure the person has used the bathroom before sitting down to eat.

Give Clear and Simple Instructions

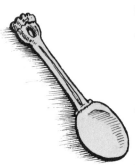

✓ Break down the eating process into simple steps. Say, "Pick up your spoon. Put some potatoes on it. Raise the spoon to your mouth."

✓ Show the person too. For example, show the person how to lift the spoon to his or her mouth by doing it yourself.

✓ Be patient and praise the person's efforts.

Plan Ahead for Meals at Restaurants

✓ If you want to eat in a restaurant, choose a well-lit familiar place where the service is fast.

✓ Plan to go before or after the meal rush. Try eating lunch at eleven o'clock instead of twelve o'clock.

✓ Don't rush the person. Eating in a restaurant should be a pleasant experience for both of you.

Problem Behaviors: Questions to Ask Your Doctor

✓ If the person you are caring for exhibits problem behaviors such as incontinence, wandering, restlessness or violent outbursts, talk with his or her doctor.

✓ Ask for a medical evaluation to check for illness or pain that could be contributing to the problem. For example, a person who is suddenly incontinent may have a urinary tract infection.

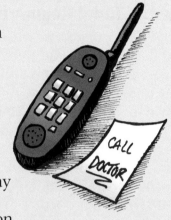

✓ Ask if the person is on medication (or combination of medications) that could be contributing to the behavior. Some medications can cause anxiety, hallucinations, paranoia, restlessness and other physical problems.

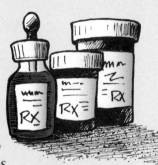

✓ If medications may be causing the problem, find out if it is possible to change medications or reduce doses.

✓ Ask if any medications may decrease or alleviate the symptoms.

✓ Have a doctor check for impaired vision and hearing. Both of these can cause confusion, increasing frustration and anger. They could signal a new medical condition.

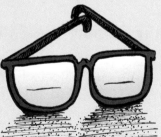

Managing Bladder and Bowel Problems

Help the Person Remember to Use the Toilet Regularly

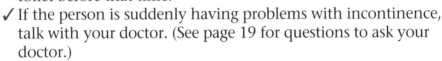

✓ Have the person use the toilet before and after meals and right before bed.
✓ Ask the person throughout the day if he or she needs to use the toilet. Or, take the person to the toilet every few hours.
✓ Look for patterns. For example, if you notice that the person has accidents after walking or eating, take him or her to the toilet before that time.
✓ If the person is suddenly having problems with incontinence, talk with your doctor. (See page 19 for questions to ask your doctor.)

Watch for Signals

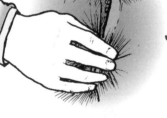

✓ Watch to see if the person pulls at his or her pants or zipper, makes faces or acts restless. These actions may signal the need to use the toilet.
✓ Learn what he or she says when needing to use the toilet. For example, some people use words from their childhood such as "tinkle."

Make Finding the Bathroom Easy

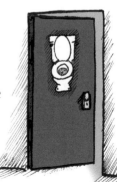

✓ Paint the bathroom door a bright color. Put a picture of a toilet on the door.
✓ Make sure the bathroom and hallway are clearly lit, especially at dusk and during the night.
✓ Remove furniture or rugs that may be blocking the way to the bathroom.

Use Simple Clothing and Protective Garments

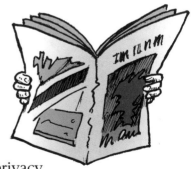

✓ Choose clothing that is loose fitting and easy to take on and off. A sweat suit is a good example.
✓ Try using Velcro tape (available at most fabric stores) to fasten clothes, instead of zippers or buttons.
✓ Buy clothing with elastic waistbands.
✓ Use adult incontinence briefs if needed. There are several different types available. If one brand is not comfortable, try another.

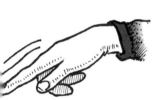

Give Clear Instructions

✓ When helping the person use the toilet, speak in a calm voice.
✓ Tell the person what to do one step at a time. For example, "Pull down your pants. Turn around."
✓ Use short, simple sentences such as, "Sit down." Try pointing or motioning with your hands too.

Help the Person Relax

✓ Recognize that the person may be embarrassed if they need help using the bathroom.
✓ Give the person a towel to fold or twist, a magazine to look at, or something else to hold while he or she is on the toilet.
✓ If it is safe to do so, give the person privacy.
✓ Have men sit down when urinating.

Make Using the Bathroom Comfortable

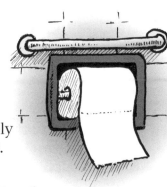

✓ Install grab bars and a raised toilet seat to make it easier for the person to get up and down.
✓ Make sure the person can sit comfortably long enough to move his or her bowels.

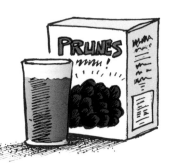

Use Fluids and Foods to Prevent Problems

✓ Give the person five to eight glasses of fluid each day to help prevent urinary track infections that can lead to incontinence.
✓ Provide plenty of liquids, fruits, vegetables and grains to help prevent constipation.
✓ Keep a food diary to pinpoint which foods cause loose bowels or constipation.

Plan for Accidents

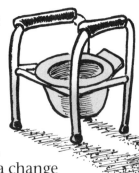

✓ Try a bedside commode at night for those who have problems getting to the toilet.
✓ Limit fluids after dinner with your doctor's approval.
✓ Use a vinyl or waterproof mattress cover under regular sheets to protect the bed.
✓ Remove any receptacle, such as a wastebasket, that could be used as a toilet.
✓ When traveling, carry supplies and bring a change of clothes. Try covering the car seat with plastic or vinyl and a towel.
✓ Remember to stay calm and keep a sense of humor when accidents happen.

Dealing with Wandering

Take Special Precautions with a Person Who Wanders

✓ If the person wanders, keep recent photos handy to assist the police in case he or she becomes lost.

✓ Have the person wear an ID bracelet or some other form of identification with his or her name and phone number. A medical alert bracelet is a good choice because it is easily noticed.

✓ Dress the person in brightly colored clothes so that he or she is easily seen.

✓ Write or sew the person's name, address and phone number in his or her clothes.

✓ Find out if your local police department, health department or Alzheimer's Association has a Wandering Program or Safe Return Program. These programs assist in locating people who are lost.

✓ Ask neighbors to notify you if they see the person out alone.

✓ If the person tries to drive when wandering, lock up the car keys or disable the car so that it won't start.

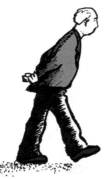

Wandering May Be OK

✓ Many people with brain impairment wander or pace. This is OK as long as the person wanders or paces in the daytime and is in a safe environment.

✓ Wandering can help relieve anxiety and restlessness. It can also be a good source of exercise.

✓ Problems may occur, however, if the person wanders away from home or wanders at night.

Take Steps to Ensure Safety

✓ Keep pathways in the home clear so the wandering person doesn't bump into things.
✓ Move low furniture that may not be easily seen.
✓ If the person wanders in the backyard, make sure that the paths are safe. Keep plants and shrubs trimmed so that they do not pose a tripping hazard. Put all yard tools and chemicals away.
✓ Make sure outside gates are secured or locked.

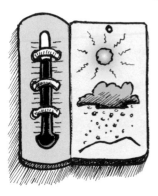

Monitor Basic Needs

✓ Sometimes people pace or wander because they are anxious.
✓ Check to see if the person is hungry, thirsty or bored.
✓ Be sure the person is not too hot or cold and does not need to use the bathroom.
✓ Make sure the person gets some type of exercise every day.
✓ Talk to a doctor to find out if medication could be causing restlessness or if medications could help the person relax.
(See page 19 for specific questions to ask your doctor.)

Redirect the Person's Attention

✓ Offer the person a favorite food or drink.
✓ Involve the person in a conversation or activity.
✓ Try joining the person as he or she wanders away from home. You can then gently guide the person to where you want him or her to be.

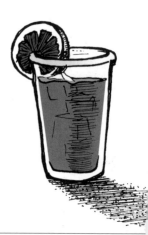

Look for Patterns

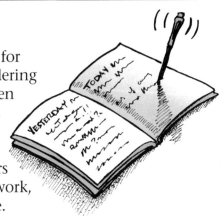

✓ Try keeping a written diary or log for several days to help identify wandering patterns. If you can figure out when and why the person wanders, you may be able to redirect his or her attention.

✓ For example, if the person wanders when he or she used to leave for work, try using a distraction at that time.

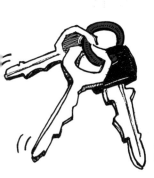

Remove Trigger Items

✓ Keep items that signal leaving the house, such as keys and coats, out of sight.

✓ Place a sign on the bathroom door so the person doesn't wander while looking for the toilet.

✓ Try covering windows or placing a black curtain over doorways to discourage the person from trying to leave.

✓ Dark, solid color mats or rugs in front of doors may discourage the person from crossing the threshold.

Be Prepared for Unexpected Wandering

✓ Lock doors and windows and put a gate across stairs. Try using locks at a height either above or below the person's eye level.

✓ Put door alarms on all doors so that you can hear if the person attempts to leave.

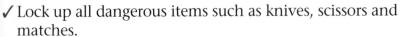

✓ Lock up all dangerous items such as knives, scissors and matches.

✓ Use soft lighting at night to reduce confusion.

Restlessness, Anxiety and Other Difficult Behaviors

Check for Physical Causes

✓ People with memory loss and confusion may become restless, anxious and agitated. They sometimes become angry or even violent.

✓ Check for comfort. See if the person needs a snack, something to drink, a sweater or to use the toilet.

✓ Check for pain, illness or constipation.

✓ Make sure the person is getting enough rest and sleep.

✓ Avoid foods and beverages with caffeine. Coffee, black tea, soft drinks and chocolate all have caffeine.

✓ Talk to your doctor about medications that may create restlessness and medications that may relieve symptoms. *(See page 19 for more about questions to ask your doctor.)*

Reduce Stress

✓ Avoid places with a lot of noise, activity and people. They can create stress.

✓ Reduce noise levels from TV and loud music. Limit the number of people around the person at one time.

✓ Notice if the person is acting lost, confused or frightened. Calmly reassure him or her.

A Special Note About Holidays

✓ For some people, large holiday gatherings create anxiety.

✓ Try celebrating in small groups or limiting the time you spend at large gatherings.

✓ If possible, leave before the person becomes anxious. If you notice early signs of anxiety, leave right away.

Offer Distractions

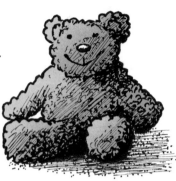

✓ Offer the person a favorite food or drink.
✓ Distract the person by starting a conversation, taking a walk, or offering a new activity.
✓ Give the person something to play with like a small ball or a stuffed animal.

Give Reassurance

✓ Offer the person affection and comfort. Tell the person that you care. Offer a hug. Hold his or her hand.
✓ Experiment with soothing objects such as a stuffed animal or a soft blanket. Having a dog or cat nearby soothes many people.

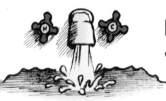

Look for Early Signs

✓ Look for signs of frustration in activities such as bathing, dressing or eating. Respond with a calm, reassuring tone.
✓ If an activity is causing anxiety, take a break and come back to it later.
✓ Remember to give yourself a break too. If you are tired, frustrated or angry, the person may react to your mood.

Evaluate Difficult Episodes

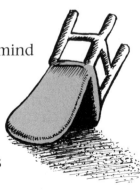

✓ After a difficult or violent episode, don't remind or blame the person. He or she may not remember what has happened.
✓ Look at what caused the problem. Is there a way to avoid the situation in the future?
✓ Mood swings sometimes happen when there is no obvious reason. Angry outbursts are not always avoidable.
✓ Remember that anger and difficult behaviors are symptoms of the disease. Don't take angry behavior personally.

Dealing with Angry Outbursts

During an Angry Outburst...

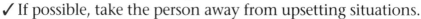

✓ Respond to anger and outbursts in a calm and direct manner.
✓ Always approach the person slowly and from the front. Make eye contact. Speak in clear, easy to understand sentences.
✓ Move five steps back from the person to see if that diffuses the anger.
✓ If possible, take the person away from upsetting situations.
✓ Avoid physically holding or restraining the person unless absolutely necessary. Restraining the person may make the situation worse.
✓ Try to distract the person with a favorite activity, food, drink or soothing object such as a stuffed toy.

Assess Danger

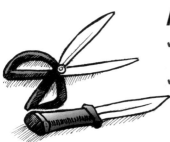

✓ Make sure the person cannot hurt him or herself. Keep sharp objects put away.
✓ If the person is physically violent, make sure you are safe. Stay out of reach or leave if necessary to avoid getting hurt.

Get Help

✓ Call family members, friends, neighbors or the person's doctor for help.
✓ If violent episodes are repeated, come up with an emergency plan to keep you both safe.
✓ If you feel your safety is threatened, call 911 or your local emergency number immediately. If you feel the person you are caring for is not safe, call 911 too.

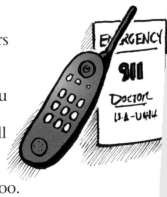

Taking Care of Yourself

Take Care of Your Needs Too

✓ Caring for a person with memory loss
and confusion can be exhausting. You
will be better able to care for someone
else if you are feeling strong and healthy.

✓ Eat regular, healthy meals. Exercise and
get plenty of rest.

✓ Get regular check ups. Have your doctor
screen you for stress and depression.

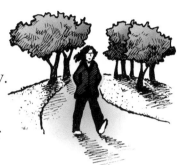

Take Breaks from Caregiving

✓ If you live full time with the person for whom you are caring,
breaks are especially important.

✓ Even a few minutes a day can help. Taking time for you can be
as simple as taking a hot bath or watching a TV program.

✓ Give yourself a treat. Buy yourself a gift, watch a sunset or go
out for a special dinner.

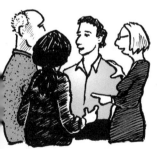

Connect with Friends and Family

✓ Don't lose contact with your friends
and family. Telephone or meet for
lunch once a week. If you have a
computer, stay in touch through email.

✓ If you feel isolated, become active in a
local community group, your church,
synagogue or other organization.

Express Your Feelings

✓ Recognize that feelings of frustration, sadness, anger and
depression are normal under the circumstances.

✓ Find a safe person – a friend, relative or another caregiver – to
talk with about your feelings.

✓ Consider talking with a counselor or therapist.

✓ Join a support group. Check with your local social services to
find out about support groups in your area.

Getting Help from Others

Caregivers Need Help

✓ Perhaps the most important – and often most difficult – part of being a caregiver is asking for help from family and friends, and using community resources.

✓ Even if asking for help is hard, find at least one resource you can use right away.

Be Prepared When Friends and Family Offer to Help

✓ Make a list of the things you need. Do you need help with cleaning or shopping? Do you need someone to give you time off by staying with the person? Do you need emotional support or someone to talk to?

✓ When friends or family members ask, "What can I do?" have them choose from the list.

✓ Be as specific as possible. Ask a friend to fix dinner or a relative to help out for an hour each week.

✓ Don't wait for a crisis. Accept help on a regular basis.

Watch for Signs of "Burnout"

✓ Ask yourself, "Am I getting enough sleep, food and exercise? Am I crying or losing my temper more than is usual for me? Do I feel all alone?" If you answer yes to any of these questions, it is time to reach out for help.

✓ Take an honest look at alcohol, tranquilizer and coffee use. Have a doctor or counselor help evaluate your use.

✓ If you feel discouraged, frustrated, trapped or overburdened, talk about it with a safe person.

✓ Seek professional help if you are thinking about suicide. Talk to your doctor or call a crisis intervention hotline.

Investigate Local Services

✓ Many communities provide respite
care and other services to assist
family caregivers and homebound
residents.

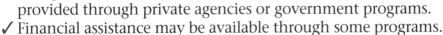
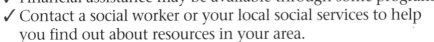

✓ Services may include adult day care,
in-home care, meal delivery,
household assistance and
transportation. Services may be
provided through private agencies or government programs.
✓ Financial assistance may be available through some programs.
✓ Contact a social worker or your local social services to help
you find out about resources in your area.

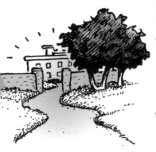

Plan for the Future

✓ Caregivers and family members will
need to plan for long term care. Find
out about nursing homes and
residential care.
✓ Even if you don't want to use a nursing
home now, it may become a necessity
in the future.

Make Legal and Financial Plans

✓ Talk with an attorney or legal aid
service about legal issues. Ask about:
• A power of attorney for legal matters.
• A power of attorney for health care
and a directive on the use of artificial
support systems (sometimes called a
living will).
• A living trust and a will.
✓ Consult with a financial planner or accountant to help
plan for future care and to help locate financial resources.

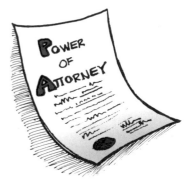

Resources

To get more information and support, you can look in your phone book for local organizations and services. Or, contact these national organizations to get more information and to locate services in your area.

Alzheimer's Disease Education and Referral Center (ADEAR)

ADEAR provides information about Alzheimer's disease and helps locate services.
English and Spanish speaking staff available.
Phone: 1-800-438-4380
www.alzheimers.org

Eldercare Locator

Provides help in locating aging services throughout the United States.
English and Spanish speaking staff available.
Phone: 1-800-677-1116
www.eldercare.gov

Family Caregiver Alliance Website

Provides free fact sheets on all aspects of caring for a person with memory loss and confusion.
www.caregiver.org

Alzheimer's Association

Provides information and referrals for those dealing with Alzheimer's disease.
Phone: 1-800-272-3900
www.alz.org

National Parkinson Foundation

Provides information and referrals for those dealing with Parkinson's disease.
Phone: 1-800-327-4545
www.parkinson.org

National Stroke Association

Provides information for stroke survivors and caregivers.
Phone: 1-800-STROKES (1-800-787-6537)
www.stroke.org